W9-DEW-982

7601 9100 346 601 1

the **Genetics** of Obesity

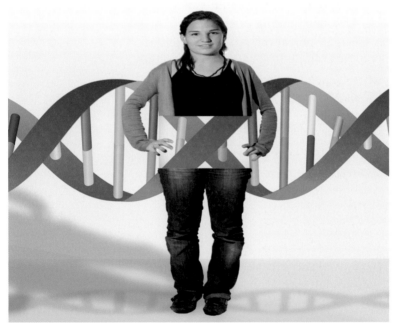

Stephanie Watson

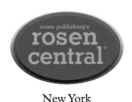

rosen publishing's
rosen central®

New York

Published in 2009 by The Rosen Publishing Group, Inc.
29 East 21st Street, New York, NY 10010

Copyright © 2009 by The Rosen Publishing Group, Inc.

First Edition

All rights reserved. No part of this book may be reproduced in any form without permission in writing from the publisher, except by a reviewer.

Library of Congress Cataloging-in-Publication Data

Watson, Stephanie, 1969–
The genetics of obesity / Stephanie Watson.
    p. cm.—(Understanding obesity)
Includes bibliographical references and index.
ISBN-13: 978-1-4042-1767-6 (library binding)
1. Obesity—Genetic aspects—Popular works. I. Title.
RC628.W48 2009
616.3'98042—dc22

                                                        2008005595

Manufactured in the United States of America

Contents

Introduction

I n 1918, an influenza epidemic swept across the United States and around the world, killing an estimated fifty million people. Epidemics of diseases such as tuberculosis, acquired immunodeficiency syndrome (AIDS), and cholera have killed millions of people throughout history.

Today, health officials are dealing with another type of epidemic. It isn't a disease, but it can cause some of the deadliest illnesses known, including heart disease, stroke, and one type of diabetes. The epidemic is obesity, and it is spreading at an alarming rate. As of 2005, 1.6 billion adults throughout the world were overweight or obese, according to the World Health Organization. In the United States, 66 percent—two out of every three people—are either overweight or obese, as reported in the 2003–2004 National Health and Nutrition Examination Survey (NHANES).

Obesity is a serious health issue, even in young people. Almost 20 percent of children ages six to eleven and 17 percent of teens are overweight, according to NHANES. If a child has one parent who is obese, then he or she is 33 percent likely to be overweight or obese. If both parents are obese, then the child is 67 percent likely to be overweight or obese.

Obesity is not a new problem, but it is getting worse. Back in the late 1970s, about 15 percent of American adults were obese. Today, that number has jumped to more than 30 percent, according to NHANES. In children ages six to eleven, obesity

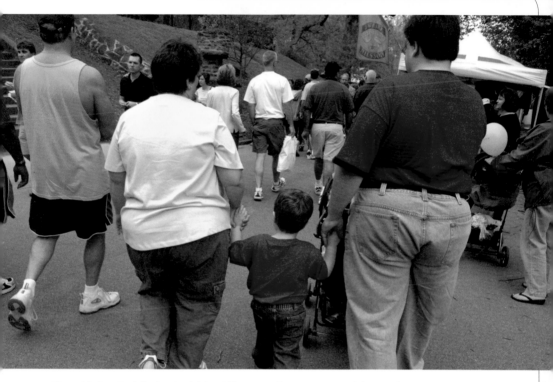

Two-thirds of adults in the United States today are overweight or obese, and that number could rise in the years to come. If both his or her parents are obese, then a child has a 67 percent chance of being overweight or obese, too.

has tripled in the past three decades. If children keep growing at this rate, the numbers of obese people will skyrocket in coming years. Using childhood obesity rates from the year 2000, researchers estimate that as many as 44 percent of American women and 37 percent of men will be obese by the year 2020, according to a study in the December 6, 2007, *New England Journal of Medicine.* That added obesity will cause 100,000 more people between the ages of thirty-five and fifty to die from heart disease.

Scientists are aware that obesity is a big problem. What they still need to figure out is *why* it is occurring.

WHY ARE PEOPLE GETTING FATTER?

The simple answer to the question of why people are gaining weight is that they are eating more and moving less than they were in years past. Dr. Susan Okie reported in her book, *Fed Up! Winning the War Against Childhood Obesity*, that women ate an average of 335 more calories per day than they did in the early 1970s, and men ate 168 more calories per day. Americans are eating more calories today, at least in part because they have greater access to high-fat, high-calorie foods—especially fast food.

In 1970, Americans spent about $6 billion on fast food, according to *Fast Food Nation*, a book written by Eric Schlosser. By 2005, Americans were spending more than $136 billion per year on fast food, *QSR Magazine* reported.

People who eat more calories than they burn with exercise store most of those calories as fat. Studies also show that Americans are exercising much less than they did a few years ago. In 1991, almost half of U.S. students took physical education class in school every day. In 2003, only 28 percent took daily gym classes, according to the Centers for Disease Control and Prevention (CDC). Americans don't exercise as much as they used to because they are too busy doing sedentary (sitting-down) activities, such as playing video games and watching television. According to the CDC, young people between the ages of eight and eighteen spend more than three hours each day just in front of the television set.

IS IT IN OUR GENES?

Food plus lack of exercise adds up to extra weight, but that is not the entire equation. Genes—the inherited instructions that tell all the cells of your body how to operate—are also proving to be an important factor in obesity.

People who claim that they have a hard time keeping off the pounds because of their genes are at least partly right. Some people do have genes that make them more likely to gain weight. However, that does not mean genes are totally to blame, or that your genes seal your fate. It turns out that obesity is a combination of who you are *and* what you do. The entire obesity equation looks something like this:

Genes + diet + exercise + other lifestyle factors = obesity

If you make good choices by watching what you eat and getting plenty of physical activity, then you can overcome your genes and stay at a normal weight.

Chapter 1

All About Obesity

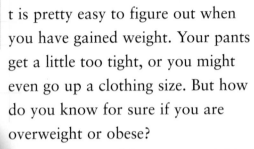

I t is pretty easy to figure out when you have gained weight. Your pants get a little too tight, or you might even go up a clothing size. But how do you know for sure if you are overweight or obese?

Being overweight means weighing more than you should for your height. That weight is not necessarily fat—it can also come from muscle, bone, or water. Obesity means having too much body fat.

Doctors have tests to pinpoint if, and by how much, a person is overweight or obese. One method requires the use of a caliper, which is a device that measures the thickness of the layer of body fat just under the skin. Another type of test sends a small, harmless amount of electrical current throughout the body. Because the current moves more quickly through parts of the body that are made up of water (such as blood and muscle), and more slowly

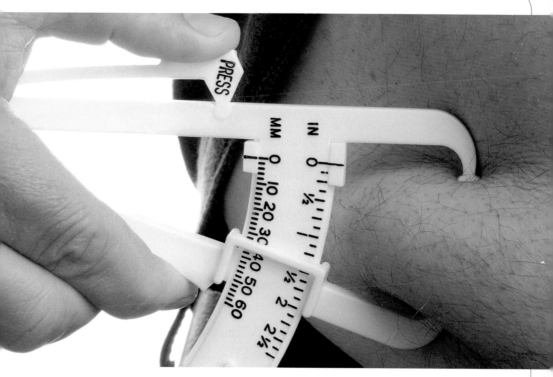

A caliper is used to determine whether a person is overweight by measuring skinfolds to help calculate the thickness of the body fat layer under the skin.

through areas made of fat, doctors can use this technique to see what percentage of body fat you have.

One of the easiest and most commonly used methods to tell whether or not a person is overweight or obese is by measuring body mass index (BMI). This simple calculation divides the person's weight in pounds by his or her height in square inches, and then multiplies that number by 703 (a conversion factor). For example, a woman who measures 5 feet 5 inches (1.65 meters) and weighs 125 pounds (57 kilograms) would have a BMI of 20.8. Here is how BMI breaks down:

- Below 18.5   Underweight
- 18.5–24.9   Normal
- 25.0–29.9   Overweight
- 30.0 and above   Obese

The BMI calculation works pretty well for adults, but it is less accurate for children because they are still growing and their body fat percentage changes as they mature. For children, doctors use a special BMI-for-age percentile. Here is how it works: Once your doctor has measured your height and weight, he or she will compare it on a chart to the height and weight of other children who are of the same age and gender. Based on your height and weight, you will fall within a certain percentile.

This is what the BMI-for-age percentile looks like:

Less than 5th percentile	Underweight
5th percentile to less than the 85th percentile	Healthy weight
85th percentile to less than the 95th percentile	Risk of overweight
95th percentile or greater	Overweight

If your BMI-for-age percentile is high, then your doctor will probably look at your family history, your diet, and your level of physical activity to find ways to lower it.

Your weight and BMI are not the only important factors to consider when it comes to your overall health. It is also important to look at where the fat is located. Women usually carry more fat in their hips and buttocks, which gives them a shape like a pear. Men carry it in their bellies, giving them an apple shape. Excess fat in general can increase your risk of getting heart disease, stroke, diabetes, and other serious diseases, but fat in the abdomen is especially dangerous.

WHY WE EAT, AND WHY WE STOP EATING

Although it might sound strange, your eating behavior operates a lot like the heating and cooling system in your home. When the temperature rises in your house, the system detects that it is getting warmer and, as a result, turns on the air conditioner. Then, when the air conditioner has been running for a while and the house gets too cold, the system turns off the air conditioner and switches back to heat. This process is called a feedback loop.

In your body, the eating feedback loop is centered in a part of your brain called the hypothalamus. The hypothalamus monitors the changes in your body and the environment, and it responds to those changes by sending orders to the pituitary gland at the base of the brain. The pituitary gland releases chemicals called hormones, which tell the body's organs to change their activities.

Depending on how much food is available, the hypothalamus increases or decreases your appetite, changes the rate at which your body burns calories, and adjusts how much energy your cells use for their normal processes. In these ways, the hypothalamus tries to make sure that you don't starve or eat too much. (As you will see, though, this isn't a perfect system.)

Messages arrive at the hypothalamus from other parts of the body, giving status reports on the amount of energy you have

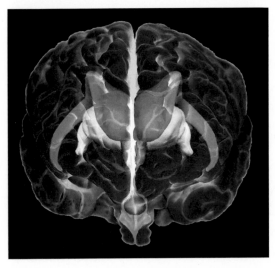

The hypothalamus (the spot highlighted in green in the center of the brain) helps control how much you eat by triggering your appetite when you're low on energy and making you feel full when you have enough energy stored up.

stored up, the level of sugar (glucose) in your blood, and the fullness of your digestive tract. The hypothalamus directs your food intake with the help of two types of nerve cells: one type of nerve cell makes the substances neuro-peptide Y (NPY) and agouti-related protein (AGRP), which increase appetite. The other type of nerve cell makes proopiomelanocortin (POMC) and cocaine- and amphetamine-regulated transcript (CART), substances that decrease appetite.

When your food stores are low, the hypothalamus releases NPY and AGRP to stimulate your appetite. After you've eaten, the hypothalamus releases POMC and CART so that you feel full and stop eating.

Hormones are also part of the hunger/fullness feedback loop. After you eat, the level of sugar (glucose) in your blood rises. In response to this rise in blood sugar, the pancreas releases a hormone called insulin, which helps the cells pull the sugar out of the blood and use it for energy. Insulin also acts on nerve cells in the hypothalamus, blocking the action of NPY so that you stop feeling hungry and triggering the action of substances that make you feel full.

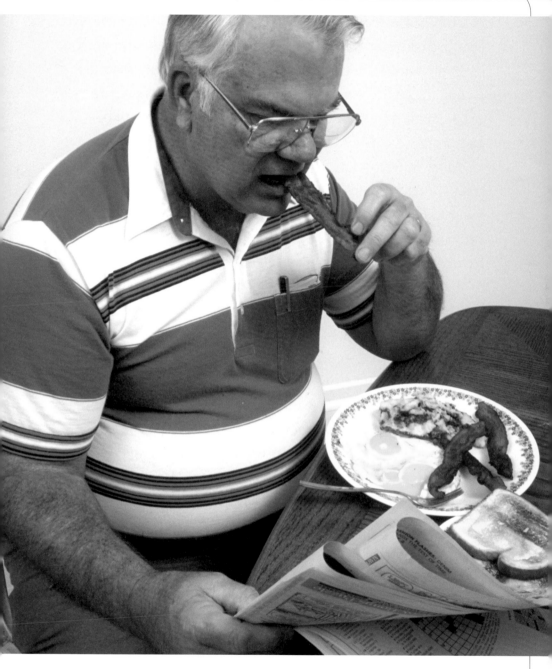

Even though people's bodies tell them when they feel full, sometimes they ignore those signals. Eating is affected by factors besides hunger; stress and happiness can also make a person want to eat.

Another hormone, leptin, makes sure the body has enough energy stored up. When you've eaten and your fat stores are high, the fat cells release leptin, which signals your brain that it is time for you to stop eating. When you don't have anything to eat, leptin levels drop, telling your brain to slow your body down and protect whatever energy stores you have left.

More hunger-related hormones are located in the digestive tract. Ghrelin is released from certain stomach cells when you are hungry. This hormone tells your hypothalamus that it is time to eat. Cholecystokinin (CCK), released by the intestines, stops the feeling of hunger after you've eaten.

If people have all of these systems telling their brain when they need to eat and when it is time to stop, how is it possible for anyone to gain weight, much less become obese? First, every person's feedback loop is slightly different. Just as each house thermostat is set at a slightly different temperature, each person's weight will hover within a specific range. This level or point at which a person's weight tends to stabilize is called a set point. Your body is in the business of keeping you alive, and that means making sure that you never starve to death. So, when you lose a few pounds by dieting and cutting back on calories, your body responds by becoming more efficient. Your metabolism slows, your cells use less energy, and you feel hungrier. That is why it is often so difficult to lose weight while on a diet.

Second, eating is influenced by other factors besides hunger. Have you ever finished an entire box of chocolates just because you were feeling stressed out, or wolfed down a piece of cake because you were having fun at a birthday party? When you eat, chemicals such as dopamine and serotonin in the reward centers

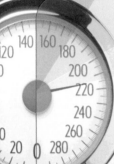

Leptin: Miracle Weight-Loss Drug?

The hormone leptin is your body's natural way of telling you to push aside that second slice of pizza and forego another helping of chocolate layer cake for dessert. Leptin tells your body when you have had enough to eat. Naturally, scientists wondered whether giving leptin to obese people might help speed their weight loss.

Research on mice seemed to suggest that leptin might treat obesity by tricking the brain into thinking that it is full. Mice that lack the genes that code for the production of leptin cannot regulate their weight and, thus, are very fat. When scientists gave these mice leptin, their body weight dropped to normal.

The problem with this research is that most obese people already make plenty of leptin. The reason they gain weight is that their brain doesn't respond correctly to the hormone, so they don't know when they are full. Instead of focusing on leptin itself, researchers are now testing weight-loss drugs that affect the entire leptin pathway that controls appetite.

of your brain give you a pleasurable feeling. Food does more than just keep you alive—it also makes you happy.

WHAT OBESITY DOES TO THE BODY

Health experts are always talking about the dangers of the "obesity epidemic." Why are they so concerned? People who are very overweight are at greater risk for many different diseases. The heavier you are, the more your risk increases. Obesity can even shorten your life. People who are obese live an average of nine fewer years than those who are of normal weight, according to a study by John R. Speakman in the August 2004 issue of the *Journal of Nutrition.*

Diseases you're more likely to get if you are obese include the following:

- **Heart disease.** People who are overweight have higher amounts of cholesterol—a fatty, wax-like substance that circulates in the blood. When you have a lot of cholesterol in your blood, it can build up inside the arteries, particularly ones that feed your heart. With less blood flowing to it, the heart has to work harder. Eventually, the heart becomes so overworked that it gets damaged and is too weak to send blood and oxygen throughout the body. People with heart disease can have a heart attack, which occurs when arteries that supply blood to the heart are entirely blocked and blood flow to the heart muscle is cut off. A stroke can also occur in people with heart disease. A stroke is the sudden blockage or bursting of a blood vessel in the brain. Without the blood and the oxygen the blood carries, the brain cells begin to die.

- **High blood pressure.** Obese people are also more likely to have high blood pressure. Blood pressure is the force at which your blood presses against the walls of the arteries as it moves from the heart to the rest of your body. In people with high blood pressure, the blood pushes against the artery walls with too much force. This increased pressure can lead to heart failure, kidney failure, a heart attack, or stroke.

- **Type 2 diabetes.** Diabetes is a condition that affects the hormone insulin, which helps the cells use the sugar from foods for energy. Type 1 diabetes occurs when the pancreas makes little or no insulin. Type 2 diabetes occurs when the pancreas makes enough (or even too much) insulin, but the cells do not respond to it. As a result, the amount of sugar in the blood rises. Type 2 diabetes is most common in people who are overweight. Type 2 diabetes used to be rare in children, but as more children are becoming overweight, the incidence of the disease is rising. Today, between 8 percent and 45 percent of new type 2 diabetes cases are in children, according to the National Heart, Lung, and Blood Institute (NHLBI). Diabetes can lead to heart disease, stroke, kidney damage, and blindness.
- **Cancer.** Many different types of cancer—including those of the colon, gallbladder, prostate, cervix, breast, uterus, and ovaries—are more common in people who are overweight.

Other conditions that are more common in people who are overweight include:

- **Gallstones.** These hard masses got their name because they look like little stones that form in the gallbladder. Gallstones can be very painful, and sometimes people who have them need surgery to have their gallbladder removed.
- **Osteoarthritis.** This disease causes the tissue that normally protects the joints (the moveable connection

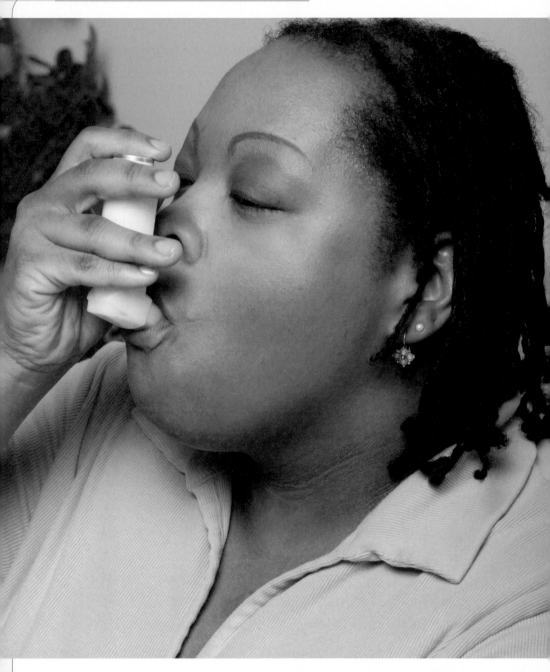

Asthma causes the airways to narrow, making it difficult to breathe. People who have asthma often use inhalers to deliver asthma medicine to their lungs and help them breathe more easily.

between your bones) to wear away. With no cushion in between them, the bones rub painfully against each other. Being overweight puts extra pressure on already weakened joints, leading to even more pain.

- **Breathing problems.** Overweight people have a higher risk of both asthma and sleep apnea. Asthma is a disease that tightens the airways, making it more difficult to breathe. Sleep apnea is a blockage of the airway that occurs at night. It causes people to stop breathing, sometimes hundreds of times each night, while they sleep. As their brain restarts breathing over and over again, people with sleep apnea keep waking up, so it is difficult for them to get a good night's sleep.

- **Emotional issues.** Obesity doesn't just affect the body. It can also lead to feelings of shame and depression. In a society where pencil-thin models and actors fill the pages of every magazine and are featured in television shows and movies, overweight people are often made to feel unattractive. It can be hard to try to fit in when you look so different from many of your peers.

Chapter 2

How People Become Obese

The most basic explanation for why people gain weight is that they eat more calories than they burn off through cell functions (such as breathing and digestion) and with exercise. If you should be eating 2,000 calories per day for your height and age but you eat 2,100 calories per day and don't add any extra exercise to your routine, then those seemingly harmless 100 extra calories per day translate into about 1 pound (.5 kg) of weight gain per month, and about 10 extra pounds (4.5 kg) of weight gain per year. That's enough extra weight to move you out of your favorite jeans and into a bigger size.

Weight gain sounds pretty simple, but there are actually other environmental and genetic factors at work. For example, some people's genes cause them to put on weight slower or faster than other people. That is why a lucky few can eat whatever they want and not gain a pound, while others say that every slice of chocolate cake they eat goes "right to their thighs."

DRUGS, DISEASE, AND WEIGHT GAIN

Some people become obese because they have an illness that causes them to gain weight. Diseases that lead to weight gain include the following:

- **Hypothyroidism.** The small, butterfly-shaped thyroid gland in the neck releases hormones that help control how quickly you burn calories (your metabolism). In people with hypothyroidism, the thyroid doesn't produce enough of its hormones, and this slows down metabolism and leads to weight gain (even though they don't eat too many calories).
- **Cushing's syndrome.** With this condition, the adrenal glands that sit on top of the kidneys produce too much of the hormone cortisol. This hormone affects metabolism and helps insulin break down sugar for energy. Having too much cortisol can cause obesity, especially in the upper part of the body.
- **Polycystic ovary syndrome (PCOS).** This disease increases the levels of male hormones in a woman's body. (Women already make very small amounts of these hormones, called androgens.) Many women with PCOS have a problem called insulin resistance. The body doesn't use insulin properly, which causes the pancreas to produce more insulin to compensate. This process leads to too much insulin in the blood. PCOS

leads to irregular menstrual periods, increased body hair, and small fluid-filled sacs (cysts) to form on the ovaries. Another symptom of PCOS is obesity.

- **Prader-Willi syndrome.** About one out of every twelve thousand babies is born with this condition, which passes to children from their parents. People who have Prader-Willi syndrome can't stop eating because the signals that normally tell the body that it is full are not working correctly. They also use calories less efficiently. There is no cure for Prader-Willi syndrome, but people who have the condition can control their weight with diet and exercise.

Several drugs can increase weight gain by stimulating the appetite, slowing the rate at which the body burns calories, or causing a person to retain water. Some of these medications are as follows:

- Antidepressants to improve mood in people who are sad or depressed
- Steroids for arthritis, allergic reactions, and certain other conditions related to the immune system
- Seizure medications for people who have epilepsy

Fortunately, doctors can prescribe alternatives to these drugs.

LIFESTYLE ISSUES

Your environment and lifestyle are very important in determining whether you gain weight or not. If you walk by a fast-food

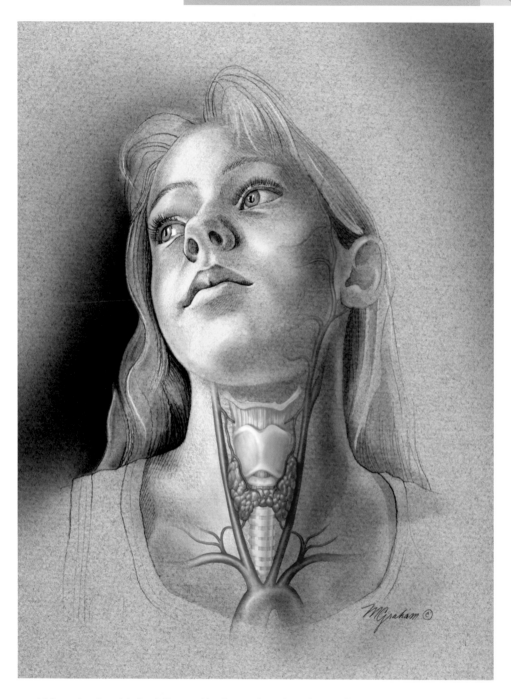

When the thyroid gland (located in the neck and made up of two lobes that lie just below your larynx) doesn't produce enough of its hormones, weight gain can result.

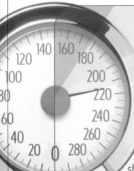

Obesity Through the Ages

Even though today's fast-food heavy and exercise-light lifestyle makes people more likely to gain weight than in years past, history shows that obesity is not a new phenomenon. Archaeologists have discovered carved figures of people with large abdomens dating from the Stone Age. Ancient peoples might have actually revered obesity. Food was so scarce that those who packed on the pounds were more likely to survive.

Eventually, though, people figured out that being overweight was not particularly healthy. Even the ancient Greeks realized the health problems that can occur with obesity, and they had some inkling that poor diet and lack of exercise led to weight gain. The Greek physician Hippocrates (460–377 BCE) wrote, "It is very injurious to health to take in more food than the constitution will bear when, at the same time, one uses no exercise to carry off this excess."

The English doctor Tobias Venner (1577–1660) was the first to use the word "obesity" to describe people who are very overweight. In his 1600 book, *Treatise*, Venner suggested bathing in the healing warm springs in the city of Bath, England, "to make slender such bodies as are too grosse."

By the 1700s, doctors started to realize that obesity was connected to diseases such as diabetes. However, it wasn't until the twentieth century that scientists really began to understand the full effects of obesity on the body.

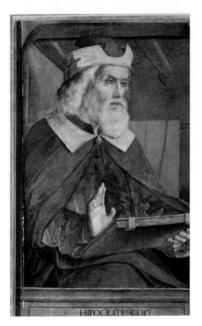

HIPOCRATI COO

The Greek physician Hippocrates understood that obesity was bad for a person's health.

restaurant every day on your way to school, then you might be more tempted to stop in and eat than you would if that restaurant was 15 miles (24 kilometers) from your home. If your mother serves cake or cookies every night after dinner, you will be more likely to want dessert than would someone whose mother never offers sweets. Other environmental factors that influence weight gain are:

- **Unhealthy food choices.** Portion sizes are getting bigger, and people are eating more calories than they need as a result. Increasingly busy lifestyles are leading more people to rely on prepackaged foods and fast foods, which are often higher in fat, sugar, and calories than fresh or homemade foods.

- **Lack of exercise.** Children today get a ride to school instead of walking and sit to watch television or play video games instead of playing outside. Watching more than two hours of TV every day can increase your risk of obesity, according to the NHLBI. While you watch TV, you are also exposed to many advertisements that try to coax you into buying unhealthy fast foods and sugary snacks.

- **Lack of sleep.** Getting a good night's sleep can not only help you perform well in school, it can also control weight gain. A 2006 study in the *International Journal of Obesity* found that grade school students who slept only eight to ten hours per night were more than three times more likely to be overweight or obese than those who slept twelve to thirteen hours per night. While you sleep, your body releases hormones that control

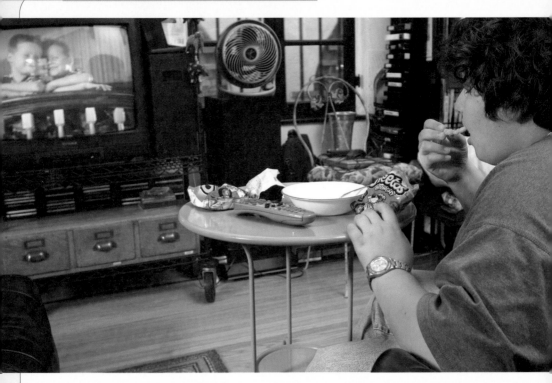

Spending more than two hours watching television every day and eating salty or sugary snacks can lead to weight gain. According to the Centers for Disease Control and Prevention, only 28 percent of U.S. students took daily gym classes in school in 2003, and young people often watch television for more than three hours each day.

your appetite and energy use. Research has found that people who don't get enough sleep have higher levels of ghrelin, the hormone that makes you feel hungry, and lower levels of leptin, the hormone that controls hunger.

- **Low income.** Studies have found that people who live in low-income areas have less access to fresh fruits and vegetables than those who live in higher-income regions. People with lower incomes also have more access to fast food and tend to buy more unhealthy processed foods because they cost less than fresh foods.

Myths and Facts

Myth: If my genes predispose me to becoming obese, there is nothing I can do to stop it.

Fact: Obesity is usually caused by a combination of genes and environmental factors. You can combat your genes and stay thin by eating a healthy diet and exercising regularly.

Myth: People who are obese eat more than people who are thin.

Fact: Although eating more calories than are appropriate for your age and height and not exercising can cause you to gain weight, other factors are involved. Genes, metabolism, diseases, and medications can all affect how much weight you gain.

Myth: People become obese because they carry a "fat gene" that causes them to gain weight.

Fact: Only a very small percentage of obesity is caused by a single gene. Most obesity stems from a combination of several genes and lifestyle habits.

Myth: Obese people are too lazy to lose weight.

Fact: Just because someone is overweight does not mean that he or she is lazy. There are many possible causes for weight gain, including certain diseases and medications.

Myth: If you are obese, you need to lose the extra weight as quickly as possible.

Fact: The healthiest and safest way to lose weight if you are obese is steadily over time by eating a healthy diet and exercising.

Chapter 3

The Gene Connection

id you know that you have a built-in blueprint that determines everything from the way you look to how your body functions? That blueprint is called your genome, and it contains the entire set of instructions, called genes, needed to run your body.

Genes are housed in the cell nucleus in structures called chromosomes, which are made up of long, twisted ladders of deoxyribonucleic acid (DNA). A gene is a section of DNA that codes for a particular protein. Each protein controls a type of cell function, which influences everything from the color of your hair to the size and shape of your ears. Genes also help determine, to some extent, whether or not you will be fat or thin. Whatever your body type, you have your parents at least partly to thank for it.

Although you might think you are a complete original, you are actually a genetic hybrid of your

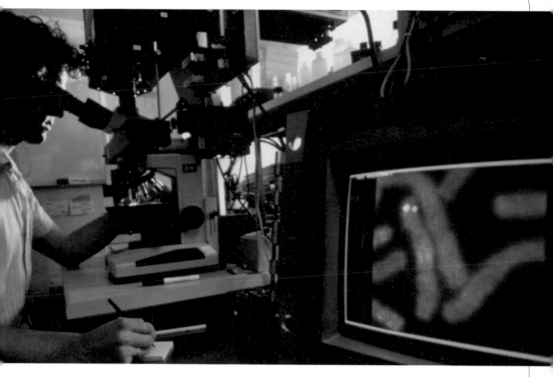

The human genome contains the set of instructions that determines everything from the color of your eyes to the shape of your body. Chromosomes are seen here in red on a monitor screen.

parents. When you were conceived, your mother's egg met your father's sperm, and their genetic material combined. You inherited half of your genes from your mother and the other half from your father. This handing down of traits is called heredity, and it is why you might have your mother's adorable dimples, but you might also have your father's much less adorable love handles.

Since the middle of the twentieth century, when an American biologist named James Watson (1928–) and a British biologist named Francis Crick (1916–2004) first identified the DNA double helix, scientists have been trying to crack the genetic code and find out how and why genes lead to disease. In 2003, a multinational research effort known as the Human Genome Project finally did crack the code. Researchers were able to identify all of the genes in the human genome—some thirty thousand of them. The next step is to hunt down the specific genes that are responsible for different conditions, including obesity.

THE STUDY OF GENES AND OBESITY

Hundreds of years ago, doctors could only guess as to why some people gained weight easily while others stayed thin. By the early twentieth century, the field of science had progressed to the point at which doctors were able to discover clues to the obesity mystery.

In the early 1900s, doctors discovered that people who had a growth called a tumor in their hypothalamus were either more or less hungry than normal. This discovery helped scientists understand that the hypothalamus plays a role in hunger and fullness. Scientists later discovered hormones in the brain and gastrointestinal tract that stimulate and stop hunger.

A big breakthrough in the study of obesity came in 1992, when scientists found a genetic defect in mice that both caused the mice to become obese and gave the mice an unusual yellow coat. Scientists named these fat, sunny-colored rodents "Yellow Obese" mice.

Because humans and mice share a similar genetic makeup, researchers used Yellow Obese mice to study human obesity. They found that the mutated gene in these mice affects the hormone leptin, which controls hunger. When scientists gave these mice leptin, they lost weight. The Yellow Obese mice showed scientists that genes can influence weight gain.

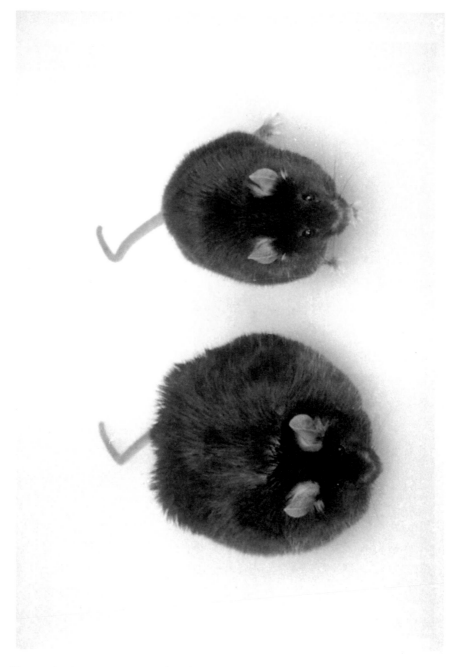

These mice have a gene mutation that causes them to gain weight. When scientists gave the hormone leptin to the mouse that appears at the top in this photograph, it lost weight.

FAT AND FAMILIES

Animals such as the Yellow Obese mouse have taught scientists a lot about obesity, but an even better way to understand human obesity is to study human genes. And the best way to hone in on obesity genes is to look at DNA from groups of people who share common genetic traits.

The most obvious source of people with similar genes is families. In the 1990s, researchers working on the San Antonio Family Heart study compared the BMI, body fat mass, and blood leptin (the hormone that makes you feel full) levels in 470 Mexican Americans from ten large families. The researchers found that family members shared similar genes that affected leptin and the amount of body fat.

One of the most important groups involved in the study of obesity is the Pima Indians, a tribe of Native Americans who have lived in southwestern Arizona for about two thousand years. The Pima Indians are fascinating to scientists because they have one of the highest rates of obesity in the world. The question is, why are they so overweight?

Many studies have found that the Pima Indians share similar genes, which adds to the evidence that heredity plays a big role in obesity. But scientists have discovered something else about this group of people. In 1994, Dr. Eric Ravussin, a visiting scientist at the National Institute of Diabetes and Digestive and Kidney Diseases (NIDDK), undertook a study comparing the Pima Indians of Arizona to their distant cousins, the Pima Indians of Mexico. He found that although the Arizona Pimas were mostly overweight, their Mexican relatives were very thin.

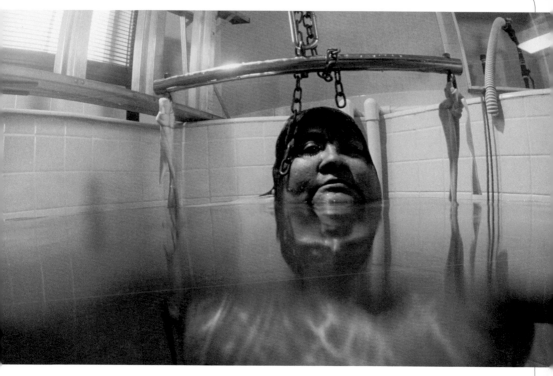

A Pima Indian has his body fat measured underwater. Scientists in Arizona are studying the Pimas to learn about obesity because this group of Native Americans has one of the highest rates of obesity in the world.

Dr. Ravussin's findings suggested that genes were not solely to blame for obesity. Diet was another important factor. While the Mexican Pimas got their food by farming the land as they had done for centuries, the Arizona Pimas had switched over to a modern American diet. The reason why these dietary changes left the two groups of Pima Indians with such different body types might have to do with an idea proposed in the 1960s by a geneticist named James Neel. He called it the "thrifty gene" theory.

The idea is that our ancestors had to hunt and forage for every bite of food they ate. Often, they starved to death because they could not find enough food. Neel proposed that a genetic change, the thrifty gene, affected metabolism and other factors to enable some people to survive on very little food. Those survivors lived to pass on their genes to future generations.

The same genetic changes that helped people to survive during harsh times work against those who have plenty of access to food today. Because their bodies are designed to horde food, the Arizona Pimas are finding it very difficult to stay thin while eating a hearty American diet.

Chapter 4

How Genes Influence Obesity

As scientists have learned from studying related groups such as the Pima Indians, obesity tends to run in families. If you have a family history of obesity, then you will be two to three times more likely to become obese than someone who does not have a family history of obesity, according to the Centers for Disease Control and Prevention (CDC). In other words, your chances of becoming overweight are much greater if one or both of your parents is heavy. Shared environmental factors, such as inactive lifestyles and eating a high-fat or unhealthy diet, also influence the tendency for obesity to run in some families.

Genes can affect your weight in all of the following ways:

- They can alter the way your body responds to the hormone leptin so

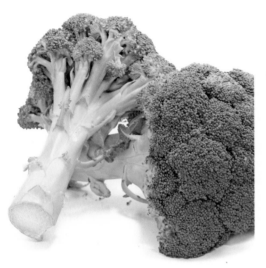

Genes can make people more likely to favor the taste of sweet foods over healthy vegetables such as broccoli.

that you feel hungry, even after you have eaten enough.

- They can affect your taste buds, making you prefer sweets and other fatty foods to healthier foods. For example, certain people's genes allow them to taste a bitter substance called PTC, which is found in broccoli and similar vegetables. If you can taste PTC, you are more likely to avoid eating these healthy vegetables.

- Genes can affect your metabolism, slowing down the rate at which your cells burn energy from food. As a result, you will store more of that energy as fat. Genes also influence where on your body you store fat (in your waist or thighs, for example).

Genes are only part of the story, though. As the case of the Pima Indians illustrates, genes set the stage for obesity, but then food intake, exercise, and other environmental influences combined decide whether or not a person will actually be overweight.

When it comes to families, all factors are at work. You inherit your parents' genes, which make you more or less likely to

An Expanding Island

The tiny island of Kosrae looks like paradise. It is located in the western portion of the Pacific Ocean just above the equator, in a group of islands known collectively as Micronesia. Kosrae is made up of white sandy beaches and lush forests, and crystal-clear blue water surrounds it.

At the turn of the twentieth century, the people on Kosrae lived off the fish, bananas, coconuts, and other fruits and vegetables that they could gather on and around the island. Although their surroundings were idyllic, the Kosraen people often struggled to find enough food to survive.

Then, after World War II (1939–1945), the United States took control of the region and began shipping in packaged foods. Life became easier for the people of Kosrae. As a result, the shape of the island's people began to change—literally.

When scientists from Rockefeller University in New York visited Kosrae in 1994, they found that more than half of the people there were obese and that 88 percent of them were overweight. The Kosraeans also had high rates of diabetes and high blood pressure, conditions that often occur in people who are overweight.

The scientists believe that the weight gain of the Kosraeans is another example of the "thrifty gene" theory. The Kosraeans' genes are designed to sustain them during harsh times. With food resources now abundant, the people of Kosrae have started to gain weight, and a lot of it. Researchers continue to study the islanders' genes to find out what clues they can provide about this startling weight gain.

become obese. Then your environment kicks in. If your mother likes to cook fried chicken and bake apple pies, and your father takes you out for fast food every other night, it will be easy for you to gain weight. On the other hand, if your parents love salads and make exercise a family routine, you will be more likely to stay thin, regardless of your genes.

LEARNING FROM TWINS

Your DNA is what makes you unique. It is different from the DNA of every other person in the world—that is, unless you have an identical twin. Only identical twins share most—if not all—of their genes. For this reason, they make ideal subjects for scientists who are studying the effects of genes versus the environment on weight gain.

In 1990, psychiatrist Albert J. Stunkard of the University of Pennsylvania conducted a study in which he compared identical twins that had been raised apart to those who had been raised together. He found that the identical twins had almost the same weight, height, and BMI, regardless of whether they were raised together or apart. Because many of the twins grew up in different environments, it appeared that genes had a lot to do with weight gain.

OBESITY GENES

Evidence is mounting that genes do influence obesity, but that doesn't mean that there is one dreaded "obesity gene." Only about 1 to 5 percent of all obesity is caused by a mutation to a single gene, according to a 2003 report by Doctors R. J. Loos

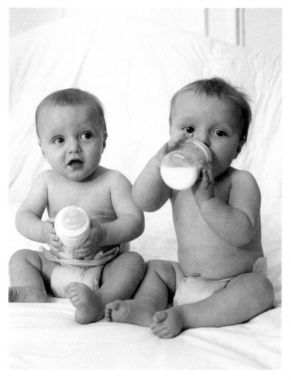

Identical twins can help researchers study the effects of genes versus environment in obesity because they share most, if not all, of their genes.

and Claude Bouchard in the *Journal of Internal Medicine*.

Most of these single-gene cases of obesity involve the melanocortin 4 receptor (MC4R) gene. This gene codes for a protein involved in the feedback loop that normally signals the hypothalamus that the body is full. When the MC4R gene is faulty, the message gets mixed up, and people keep eating and eating because they think they are still hungry.

In 2003, researcher Stephen O'Rahilly and his colleagues found the MC4R mutation in about 6 percent of the obese people they studied. They also found that children with the MC4R gene mutation ate three times as much breakfast cereal as those who did not have the mutation.

Four years later, researchers in England discovered another major obesity gene. After reviewing genetic information taken from more than thirty-eight thousand children and adults in the United Kingdom and throughout Europe, the researchers

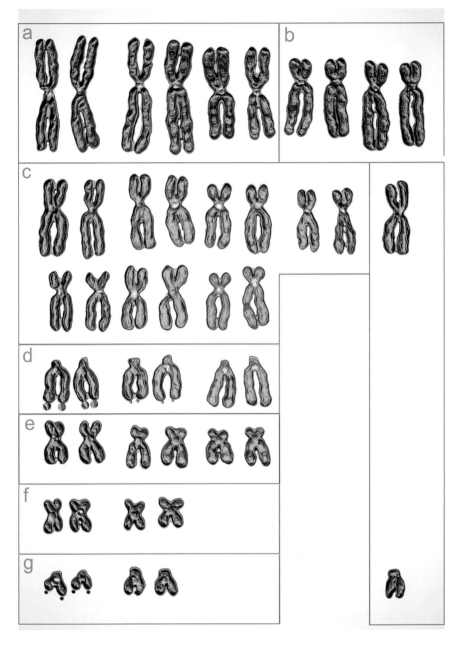

The human karyotype is a picture of the chromosomes in a cell that scientists can use to check for abnormalities. The example shown here is a boy's karyotype, showing the XY sex chromosome in the twenty-third pair. A girl's karyotype would show the sex chromosome as XX.

announced they had found a variation of a gene that they say increases the risk for obesity by 67 percent.

People who had this gene variation, known as FTO (fat mass and obesity-associated gene), had more body fat and a higher BMI than those who didn't have the gene variation, the researchers reported in the April 12, 2007, issue of *Science* magazine. The gene also appears to increase the risk for type 2 diabetes. Scientists think that this one gene might be responsible for more than 20 percent of all obesity. The next step for researchers is to find out exactly how the FTO gene affects weight gain.

"Skinny Genes"

If genes can cause some people to get fat, then it would make sense that they can also keep certain people thin. In 2007, scientists announced they had found an actual "skinny" gene.

A graduate student named Winifred Doane stumbled across this gene, which she named adipose, while studying fruit flies fifty years ago at Yale University. She noticed that fruit flies that had this gene were much skinnier than those that did not have the gene.

Fast-forward a half-century, where researchers at the University of Texas Southwestern Medical Center began testing the effects of this "skinny" gene on other kinds of animals. When they inserted the gene in mouse embryos, the mice that developed had about one-third the body weight of normal mice.

The researchers say that it is too early to turn their findings into any kind of cure for obesity. However, their research has given them greater insight into the mysteries of weight gain.

Unable to Stop Eating

In 1997, scientists at the University of Cambridge in England reported on an unusual case: Two cousins in a Pakistani family—a boy and a girl—were severely obese. At age nine, the girl weighed 200 pounds (91 kg). At just two years old, the boy weighed 65 pounds (29.5 kg). The cousins were so overweight that they could barely move.

Both children came from average-sized parents and were of normal weight when they were born. Yet, once they started eating, they just could not stop. The children's hunger was so insatiable that their parents had to lock the kitchen cabinets at night to keep them from eating everything in sight. Sometimes the little boy and girl were so desperate for food that they would dig through the garbage looking for scraps.

When doctors examined the children, they found a very rare genetic mutation that prevented their bodies from making leptin. Without this hormone, the hypothalamus never received the signal that these children were full, and, as a result, their appetites never ceased. When doctors gave the children leptin injections, their weight dropped. Eventually, both cousins got down to normal weights.

Leptin would seem from this research like a miracle cure for obesity, but, unfortunately, most obese people make enough leptin. It is just that their bodies are unable to respond to it properly, or that they ignore this signal and continue to consume too many calories.

GENES THAT INFLUENCE OBESITY

These are just a few of the genes scientists have discovered that can affect obesity:

Gene	What It Controls
Apolipoprotein-B (APOB)	BMI, percent body fat, abdominal fat
Beta-3-adrenergic receptor (ADRB3)	Weight gain, BMI, fat mass, waist size
Glucocorticoid receptor (GRL)	Abdominal fat, BMI, leptin
Leptin receptor (LEPR)	Percent body fat, BMI, abdominal fat, weight loss
Neuromedin beta (NMB)	Eating behavior, feeling full
Propiomelanocortin (POMC)	Leptin, early-onset obesity
6-n-propylthiouracil (PROP)	Taste preference
Peroxisome proliferative activated receptor (PPAR)	Fat metabolism

GENES WORKING TOGETHER

Most of the time, several genes work together to affect how much food people eat, how much energy they use, how hungry they are, what foods they like to eat, how quickly they feel full, and how well their cells burn energy (metabolism). All these factors can contribute to obesity.

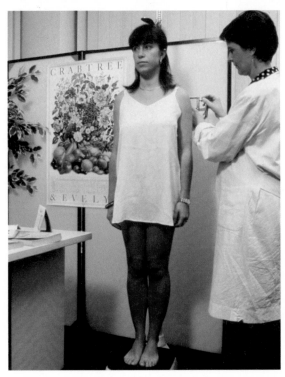

This nutritionist is measuring a patient's skinfolds by using a caliper during a counseling session. Genes are part of the reason why some people gain weight quickly, while others stay slim.

Researchers believe there may be as many as four hundred different gene variations that, when combined with factors in the environment, influence obesity. Because everyone has unique genes and is exposed to different environments, a group of people can eat exactly the same diet and gain weight in different ways. Finding the genes that affect weight gain can help scientists understand the causes of obesity and might one day lead to new treatments for the condition.

Chapter 5

Overcoming Genes

When looking at the connection between genes and obesity, it is important to remember that genes are not destiny. Just because you might have inherited your mother's tendency to gain weight doesn't mean that you *will* gain weight. You can overcome your genes through good habits, such as watching your diet and getting regular exercise. It is important to establish these good habits early, while you are still young, so that you can minimize the effects of your genes on your weight.

FOODS TO EAT

Your diet should be lean and mean. Go heavy on the fruits and vegetables, and light on the meats and sweets. Trim the fats and skimp on the carbohydrates.

According to the MyPyramid plan from the U.S. Department of

Agriculture (USDA), your daily diet should look similar to the following:

Food Group	How Much You Need Each Day	Good Sources
Whole grains	5–7 ounces	Oatmeal, brown rice, whole-wheat bread and pasta
Vegetables	2–3 cups	Broccoli, spinach, squash, sweet potatoes
Fruits	1½–2 cups	Apples, bananas, oranges, strawberries, grapes, raisins
Milk	3 cups	Low-fat or skim milk, yogurt, cheese
Meat & Beans	5 ounces	Lean beef, pork or chicken, fish, eggs, beans, peas, nuts
Oils	5 teaspoons	Nuts, olives, avocados, vegetable oil

Source: The U.S. Department of Agriculture

FOODS TO AVOID

High-fat, sugary foods will make you gain weight and will clog your arteries. Limit or avoid foods that are heavy in these unhealthy ingredients:

- **Saturated fat:** meat, whole milk, ice cream, coconut oil, and palm oil (get less than 10 percent of your total daily calories from saturated fats)

- Trans fat: any foods made with hydrogenated oils, including margarine, cookies and other baked goods, and fried foods (get less than 1 percent of your daily calories from trans fats)
- Cholesterol: egg yolks, liver and other organ meats, shrimp, and whole-milk products
- Sugar and high-fructose corn syrup: sweetened fruit drinks, soft drinks, and desserts
- Salt: processed lunch meats, some canned foods, hot dogs, and potato chips

TIPS FOR HEALTHIER EATING

Eating better is easier than you might think. You won't have to give healthy eating a second thought if you incorporate these simple tips into your daily routine:

- Read the labels. Before you grab cookies off the supermarket shelf, see what they are made of. Put back any foods that are high in fat, salt, sugar, and calories. Instead, stock up on items that are packed with nutrition, such as fruit, nuts, whole-wheat crackers, and yogurt.
- Ban fried foods. Grill, steam, bake, or broil your food instead of frying it to save on fat and calories.
- Watch your portions. Never grab a bag of potato chips and eat it in front of the TV because you can end up mindlessly munching your way to the bottom of the bag. Consider this: One serving of baked potato chips contains 3 grams of fat and 110 calories—but that serving

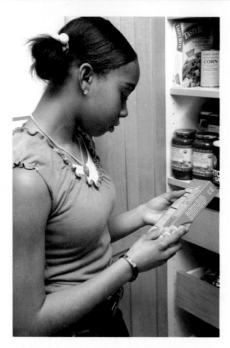

Before you buy food at the store, read the labels for the nutritional content. Any product that is high in sugar, saturated and trans fats, and sodium (salt) is one to put back on the shelf.

is just twenty-eight potato chips! If you eat the whole ten-serving bag, you will wind up ingesting 1,200 calories and 30 grams of fat, not to mention 2,000 milligrams of salt.

- **Keep a diary.** A hot-fudge sundae and large order of fries look a lot worse when you have to account for them on paper. Try writing down everything you eat during the month. Use your food diary as an incentive to stick to your healthy eating plan.

GET MOVING

Eating right isn't the only way to stay at a healthy weight. You also need to exercise. Keeping in shape has so many benefits: it lowers your risk of diabetes and heart disease, strengthens your muscles, protects your bones, gives you strength and energy, and can even help you feel less stressed out.

Aim for at least sixty minutes of moderate-intensity exercise on most, if not all, days of the week. Some examples of physical activity include the following:

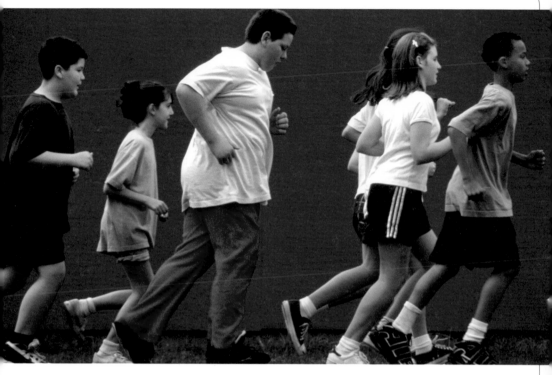

Running with your friends is just one way to get the recommended sixty minutes of exercise you need each day. If you have not had a regular running routine, start out slowly and then build up to your goal. Remember to make healthy and safe decisions about exercise.

- Walking
- Riding your bike
- Inline skating
- Dancing
- Swimming
- Taking an aerobics class
- Playing tennis

If your schedule is so packed with school, homework, and activities that you can't get in a full hour of exercise, then

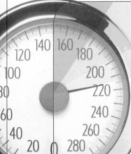

Ten Great Questions to Ask a Doctor

1. Does obesity run in my family?

2. If I carry the genes for obesity, will I definitely become obese?

3. What is my BMI, and what does it mean?

4. Why am I overweight when my parents and siblings are thin?

5. What other factors contribute to obesity?

6. What are the health risks to being overweight?

7. Do I need to lose weight?

8. What are the best ways for me to lose weight?

9. Are there certain foods I should eat, or avoid, based on my genes?

10. Even if I eat right and exercise, is there a chance that I will still gain weight?

squeeze in a few minutes whenever you find time. You could take the stairs a few extra times at home, walk the long way to school, or rake leaves in your backyard. Every little bit counts.

Also, don't feel as though you have to run a marathon within a week of starting your exercise program. Start slowly and gradually build up your routine. You might work out for just fifteen minutes the first day and then add five minutes at a time to your exercise program as you become more comfortable with it. Reward yourself for achieving your goals by buying a CD that you have been wanting or by treating yourself to a movie.

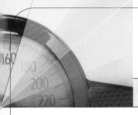

Glossary

body mass index (BMI) A measure of weight in relation to height.

caliper A device that measures the thickness of the layer of body fat under the skin to determine obesity.

chromosomes Structures found in the cell nucleus that contain the genetic material DNA.

deoxyribonucleic acid (DNA) The double-stranded material inside the cell nucleus that carries genetic information.

diabetes A disease in which a person's body either does not make insulin (a hormone needed for the cells to use sugar from foods) or does not use it properly.

genes Segments of DNA that carry the instructions for making proteins.

heart attack A blockage of blood flow to the heart that can severely damage the heart.

heredity The passing of traits from parents to their children.

hypothalamus The part of the brain that helps regulate temperature, sleep, and food intake.

insulin A hormone produced by the pancreas that helps the cells use the sugar from food as energy.

karotype A picture of the chromosomes that scientists can use to check for abnormalities.

leptin A hormone that helps control appetite.

metabolism The processes by which the cells use energy.

mutation A change in a gene that can lead to disease.

obesity Having too much body fat and a BMI above 30.

overweight A condition of weighing more than you should based on your height.

sleep apnea A condition in which one's breathing is interrupted many times while asleep. It can be caused by an obstruction, such as enlarged tonsils, in the passageway connecting the throat and nose. Being overweight can affect the development of sleep apnea.

stroke A blockage in the blood flow to the brain, which can cause part of the brain to not get enough oxygen.

trans fat An unhealthy type of fat found in fried foods, baked goods, and processed foods. Eating too much trans fat can increase your risk of heart disease.

type 2 diabetes A disease that occurs when the body can no longer use insulin properly. It is more common in people who are overweight.

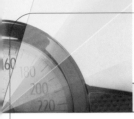

American Dietetic Association
120 South Riverside Plaza, Suite 2000
Chicago, IL 60606-6995
(800) 877-1600
Web site: http://www.eatright.org
This group is made up of about 67,000 food and nutrition experts who encourage healthy eating and help combat the problem of obesity.

Canadian Obesity Network
Royal Alexandra Hospital
Room 102, Materials Management Centre
10240 Kingsway Avenue
Edmonton, AB T5H 3V9
· Canada
Web site: http://www.obesitynetwork.ca/home.aspx
The more than one thousand health professionals who make up the Canadian Obesity Network look for solutions to Canada's growing obesity problem.

The Endocrine Society
8401 Connecticut Avenue, Suite 900
Chevy Chase, MD 20815
(888) 363-6274
Web site: http://www.endo-society.org
This organization is involved in the study and treatment of endocrine system disorders, including obesity.

The Obesity Society

8630 Fenton Street, Suite 918

Silver Spring, MD 20910

(301) 563-6526

Web site: http://www.obesity.org

The Obesity Society is dedicated to the study of obesity, including its causes
and possible treatments.

Public Health Agency of Canada

130 Colonnade Road

A. L. 6501H

Ottawa, ON K1A 0K9

Canada

http://www.phac-aspc.gc.ca/new_e.html

This official government agency works to keep Canadians healthier.

Weight-Control Information Network

1 WIN Way

Bethesda, MD 20892-3665

(877) 946-4627

Web site: http://win.niddk.nih.gov/about/index.htm

This arm of the National Institutes of Health gives consumers information
about how to control their weight and prevent obesity.

Web Sites

Due to the changing nature of Internet links, Rosen Publishing
has developed an online list of Web sites related to the subject of
this book. This site is updated regularly. Please use this link to
access the list:

http://www.rosenlinks.com/uno/geob

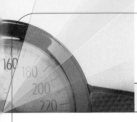

For Further Reading

Abramowitz, Melissa. *Diseases and Disorders—Obesity.*
Detroit, MI: Lucent Books, 2004.

Akers, Charlene. *Obesity.* Farmington Hills, MI: Gale Group,
2000.

Daly, Melissa. *Weighing In: How to Understand Your Body,
Lose Weight, and Live a Healthier Lifestyle.* New York, NY:
Amulet Books, 2006.

Gordon, Melanie Apel. *Let's Talk About Being Overweight.*
New York, NY: Rosen Publishing, 2003.

Harmon, Daniel E. *Obesity* (Coping in a Changing World).
New York, NY: Rosen Publishing, 2007.

Heller, Tanya, M.D. *Overweight: A Handbook for Teens and
Parents.* Jefferson, NC: McFarland & Company, 2005.

Hunter, William. *How Genetics and Environment Shape Us:
The Destined Body* (Obesity: Modern-Day Epidemic).
Philadelphia, PA: Mason Crest Publishers, 2006.

Loonin, Meryl. *Overweight America.* Detroit, MI: Lucent
Books, 2006.

Tecco, Betsy Dru. *Food for Fuel: The Connection Between Food
and Physical Activity.* New York, NY: Rosen Publishing, 2005.

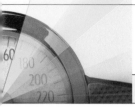

Bibliography

Bray, George, and Claude Bouchard. *Handbook of Obesity: Etiology and Pathophysiology.* New York, NY: Marcel Dekker, Inc., 2004.

Centers for Disease Control and Prevention. "About BMI for Children and Teens." May 22, 2007. Retrieved October 17, 2007 (http://www.cdc.gov/nccdphp/dnpa/bmi/childrens_BMI/about_childrens_BMI.htm).

Centers for Disease Control and Prevention. "Contributing Factors." May 22, 2007. Retrieved October 10, 2007 (http://www.cdc.gov/nccdphp/dnpa/obesity/contributing_factors.htm).

Centers for Disease Control and Prevention. "Frequently Asked Questions." May 22, 2007. Retrieved October 10, 2007 (http://www.cdc.gov/nccdphp/dnpa/obesity/faq.htm).

Centers for Disease Control and Prevention. "Obesity and Genetics: A Public Health Perspective." September 10, 2007. Retrieved October 10, 2007 (http://www.cdc.gov/genomics/training/perspectives/files/obesedit.htm).

Centers for Disease Control and Prevention. "Overweight and Obesity." May 22, 2007. Retrieved October 10, 2007 (http://www.cdc.gov/nccdphp/dnpa/obesity/).

Chaput, J. P., M. Brunet, and A. Tremblay. "Relationship Between Short Sleeping Hours and Childhood Overweight/Obesity: Results from the 'Québec en Forme' Project." *International Journal of Obesity*, July 2006, Volume 30, pp. 1,080–1,085.

Corella, D., C. Q. Lai, S. Demissie, L. A. Cupples, A. K. Manning, K. L. Tucker, and J. M. Ordovas. "APOA5 Gene Variation Modulates the Effects of Dietary Fat Intake on Body Mass Index and Obesity Risk in the Framingham Heart Study." *Journal of Molecular Medicine*, February 2007, Volume 85, Number 2, pp. 119–128.

Diliberti, Nicole, Peter L. Bordi, Martha T. Conklin, Liane S. Roe, and Barbara J. Rolls. "Increased Portion Size Leads to Increased Energy Intake in a Restaurant Meal." *Obesity Research*, 2004, Volume 12, pp. 562–568.

Duncan, David Ewing. "Wired to Eat." *Technology Review*, July 2005, Volume 108, Number 7, pp. 52–59.

Farooqi, I. Sadaf, Julia M. Keogh, Giles S. H. Yeo, Emma J. Lank, Tim Cheetham, and Stephen O'Rahilly. "Clinical Spectrum of Obesity and Mutations in the Melanocortin 4 Receptor Gene." *New England Journal of Medicine*, March 20, 2003, Volume 348, Number 12, pp. 1,085–1,095.

Farooqi, I. Sadaf, Giles S. H. Yeo, Julia M. Keogh, Shiva Aminian, Susan A. Jebb, Gary Butler, Tim Cheetham, and Stephen O'Rahilly. "Dominant and Recessive Inheritance of Morbid Obesity Associated with Melanocortin 4 Receptor Deficiency." *Journal of Clinical Investigation*, July 2000, Volume 106, Number 2, pp. 271–279.

Frayling, Timothy M., Nicholas J. Timpson, Michael N. Weedon, Eleftheria Zeggini, Rachel M. Freathy, Cecilia M. Lindgren, John R. B. Perry, et al. "A Common Variant in the FTO Gene is Associated with Body Mass Index and Predisposes to Childhood and Adult Obesity." *Science*, April 12, 2007, Volume 316, Number 5826, pp. 889–894.

Haslam, D. "Obesity: A Medical History." *Obesity Reviews*, 2007, Volume 8 (Supplement 1), pp. 31–36.

Loos, R. J., and C. Bouchard. "Obesity: Is It a Genetic Disorder?" *Journal of Internal Medicine*, November 2003, Volume 254, Number 5, pp. 401–425.

Martinez, J. A., M. S. Corbalan, A. Sanchez-Villegas, L. Forga, A. Marti, and M. A. Martinez-Gonzalez. "Obesity Risk Is Associated with Carbohydrate Intake in Women Carrying the Gln27Glu Beta2-adrenoceptor Polymorphism." *Journal of Nutrition*, 2003, Volume 133, Number 8, pp. 2,549–2,554.

Mencimer, Stephanie. "Why We Eat: The Science of Obesity." *Washington Monthly*, October 2002, Volume 34, Number 10, pp. 50–52.

Mishori, Ranit. "Bottomless Hunger; It's Not a Lack of Willpower That Drives Her to Eat Constantly. It's Her Genes. What Can Obesity Experts Learn from Her?" *Washington Post*, November 2, 2004, p. F01.

National Heart Lung and Blood Institute. "Overweight and Obesity." Retrieved October 10, 2007 (http://www.nhlbi.nih.gov/health/dci/Diseases/obe/obe_all.html).

Newell, Astrid, Amy Zlot, Kerry Silvey, and Kiley Ariail. "Addressing the Obesity Epidemic: A Genomics Perspective." *Prevention of Chronic Disease*, April 2007. Retrieved October 10, 2007 (http://www.cdc.gov/pcd/issues/2007/apr/06_0068.htm).

Ochoa, M. C., A. Marti, C. Azcona, M. Chueca, M. Oyarzabal, R. Pelach, et al. "Gene-Gene Interaction Between PPAR Gamma 2 and ADR Beta 3 Increases Obesity Risk in Children and Adolescents." *International Journal of Obesity and*

Related Metabolic Disorders, 2004, Volume 28, Supplement 3, pp. S37–41.

Okie, Susan. *Fed Up! Winning the War Against Childhood Obesity*. Washington, DC: Joseph Henry Press, 2005.

"The QSR 50: The Game in '05." *QSR Magazine*. Retrieved March 30, 2007 (http://www.qsrmagazine.com/reports/qsr50/2006/part1-3.phtml#).

Randerson, James. "Some of Us Are Born to Binge." *New Scientist*, March 29, 2003, Volume 177, Issue 2388, p. 16.

Ravussin, E., M. E. Valencia, J. Esparza, P. H. Bennett, and L. O. Schultz. "Effects of a Traditional Lifestyle on Obesity in Pima Indians." *Diabetes Care*, September 1994, Volume 17, Issue 9, pp. 1,067–1,074.

Schlosser, Eric. *Fast Food Nation*. Boston, MA: Houghton Mifflin Company, 2001.

Speakman, John R. "Obesity: The Integrated Roles of Environment and Genetics." *Journal of Nutrition*, August 2004, Volume 134, Issue 8S, pp. 2,090S–2,105S.

Stunkard A. J., J. R. Harris, N. L. Pedersen, and G. E. McClearn. "The Body-Mass Index of Twins Who Have Been Reared Apart." *New England Journal of Medicine*, 1990, Volume 322, Number 21, pp. 1,483–1,487.

Suh, Jae Myoung, Daniel Zeve, Renee McKay, Jin Seo, Zack Salo, Robert Li, Michael Wang, and Jonathan M. Graff. "Adipose Is a Conserved Dosage-Sensitive Antiobesity Gene." *Cell Metabolism*, September 2007, Volume 6, pp. 195–207.

Tholin, S., F. Rasmussen, P. Tynelius, J. Karlsson. "Genetic and Environmental Influences on Eating Behavior: The Swedish Young Male Twins Study." *American Journal of Clinical Nutrition*, 2005, Volume 81, Number 3, pp. 564–569.

Trust for America's Health. "F as in Fat: How Obesity Policies Are Failing in America, 2007." August 27, 2007. Retrieved October 14, 2007 (http://healthyamericans.org/reports/obesity2007).

Wardle, J., C. Guthrie, S. Sanderson, L. Birch, and R. Plomin. "Food and Activity Preferences in Children of Lean and Obese Parents." *International Journal of Obesity and Related Medical Disorders*, 1998, Volume 22, Number 8, pp. 758–764.

Weight-Control Information Network. "Understanding Adult Obesity." March 2006. Retrieved October 10, 2007 (http://win.niddk.nih.gov/publications/understanding.htm).

World Health Organization. "Obesity and Overweight." September 2006. Retrieved October 22, 2007 (http://www.who.int/mediacentre/factsheets/fs311/en/index.html).

World Health Organization. "Report on the Global AIDS Epidemic 2006." May 2006. Retrieved October 26, 2007 (http://www.unaids.org/en/HIV_data/2006GlobalReport/default.asp).

Zenk, S. N., A. J. Schulz, B. A. Israel, S. A. James, S. Bao, and M. L. Wilson. "Fruit and Vegetable Access Differs by Community Racial Composition and Socioeconomic Position in Detroit, Michigan." *Ethnicity & Disease*, Winter 2006, Volume 16, Number 1, pp. 275–280.

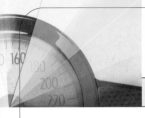

Index

About the Author

Stephanie Watson is a writer and editor based in Atlanta, Georgia. She has written or contributed to more than a dozen health and science books, including *Endometriosis, Encyclopedia of the Human Body: The Endocrine System, The Mechanisms of Genetics: An Anthology of Current Thought,* and *Science and Its Times.* Her work has been featured in several health and wellness Web sites, including Rosen's Teen Health & Wellness database.

Photo Credits

Cover, p. 1 (DNA) © www.istockphoto.com/Julia Polishchuk, (Girl) © www.istockphoto.com/Claudia Dewald; p. 5 © Robin Nelson/Photo Edit; p. 9 © www.istockphoto.com/Jim DeLillo; p. 12 © Zephyr/Photo Researchers; p. 13 © Tony Freeman/Photo Edit; pp. 18, 44 © Custom Medical Stock Photo; p. 23 © Michele S. Graham/Photo Researchers; p. 24 © Scala/Art Resource; p. 26 © Bill Aron/Photo Edit; pp. 29, 33 © Peter Menzel/Photo Researchers; p. 31 © AP Photos; p. 36 Shutterstock.com; p. 39 © Paul Whitehill/Photo Researchers; p. 40 © Cavallini/Custom Medical Stock Photo; p. 48 © David Young-Wolff/Photo Edit; p. 49 © Will Hart/Photo Edit.

Editor: Kathy Kuhtz Campbell; Photo Researcher: Marty Levick